CALISTHENICS WORKOUT GUIDE

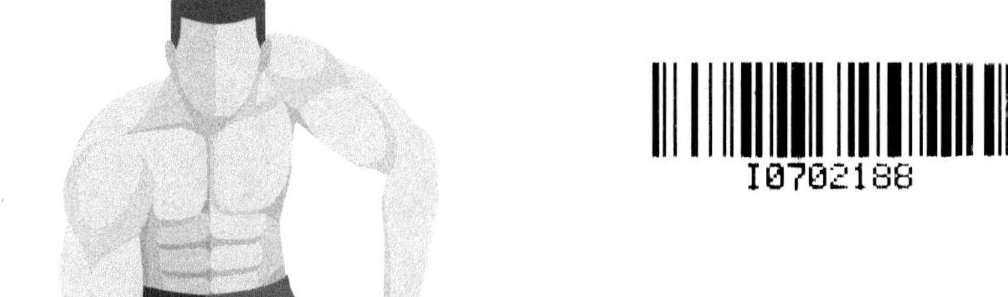

Bodyweight Exercises and Training Routines for Burning Fat, Building Muscle, Improving Strength and Losing Weight Through Pushups, Pullups, Squats, Dips and More

Troy Vhodes

Table of Contents

Warm-up and Cool-down Routines:
   - Importance of a thorough warm-up.
   - Cooling down for recovery.

Chapter 4: Structuring Your Workouts
    Sample Workout Programs:
   - Full-body routines for different fitness goals.
   - How to balance strength and cardio.

Adding Intensity: Weighted Calisthenics:
   - Incorporating resistance for continued progress.

Chapter 5: Nutrition and Diet Tips
    Eating for Success:
      - Nutritional guidance to complement calisthenics training.
   - Balancing macronutrients and hydration.

Chapter 6: Mindset and Motivation
 Building a Positive Mindset:
   - The role of mental resilience in fitness.
   - Staying motivated on the journey.

Chapter 7: Avoiding Common Pitfalls
 Common Mistakes to Avoid:
   - Preventing injuries and setbacks.
   - Troubleshooting plateaus.

Conclusion

Introduction

In the realm of fitness, we often find ourselves on a quest for the ideal workout regimen—one that not only challenges our bodies but transforms us from within. Imagine a journey where every pushup, every squat, and every pullup brings you closer to a version of yourself you've always aspired to be. This is not just a workout guide; it's a roadmap to unlocking your true potential through the transformative power of calisthenics.

Let me take you back to a time when I too grappled with the limitations of traditional fitness routines. I was searching for something more, something that would not just sculpt my physique but ignite a passion for strength and resilience. It was then that I stumbled upon calisthenics, a revelation that changed the course of my fitness journey.

Picture this: A realm where you are not confined by gym walls or beholden to expensive equipment. Instead, you harness the power within, leveraging your own body weight to sculpt a body that radiates strength and vitality. Calisthenics is more than just a workout; it's a celebration of what the human body is capable of achieving.

As the great Aristotle once said, "Excellence is an art won by training and habituation." This rings especially true in the world of calisthenics, where each movement is a brushstroke, crafting a masterpiece of strength and agility.

Did you know that calisthenics has been the secret weapon of athletes, trainers, and celebrities alike? It's not just a workout; it's a lifestyle embraced by those seeking not only physical prowess but a holistic approach to health and fitness.

Now, here's a question that might resonate with you: What if you could sculpt the body you desire in just 30 minutes a day, without the need for expensive equipment or a gym membership? The answer lies within the pages of this guide.

In the chapters that follow, we'll dive deep into the world of calisthenics, exploring its unique advantages over other training methods. We'll share stories of triumph over fitness struggles, unveil the secrets of effective bodyweight training, and provide you with a roadmap to your own success.

Expect more than just a workout routine; anticipate a transformation, a journey that will not only reshape your body but redefine your understanding of fitness. Are you ready to embark on this extraordinary adventure? Turn the page and let the calisthenics journey begin. Your body, your strength, your story, start sculpting them today.

Chapter 1
Understanding Calisthenics
What is Calisthenics?

Alright, buckle up, we're diving into the world of calisthenics! So, what in the world is calisthenics? Picture this: a workout so dynamic, so liberating, it feels like your body is throwing a celebration. That, my friend, is the essence of calisthenics.

Let's Define the Game-Changer:

Calisthenics isn't your run-of-the-mill workout; it's your body becoming the gym. No fancy machines, no overpriced memberships just you, your determination, and a whole lot of movement. In a nutshell, it's fitness unleashed, untamed, and utterly invigorating.

Unraveling the Calisthenics Tale:

Now, let's go back in time a bit. The history of calisthenics is like a tapestry woven with threads of strength, agility, and rebellion against the mundane. It's been the silent force behind warriors, athletes, and everyday superheroes, quietly sculpting bodies into feats of physical artistry.

Calisthenics vs. the Usual Suspects:

Before we go any further, let's clear the air. Calisthenics isn't just a workout; it's a movement (literally). It's not about mindlessly lifting weights or endlessly pounding the pavement. Calisthenics is the cool kid on the block, defying gravity and challenging the norms of conventional exercise.

Now, imagine your body as a canvas, and each calisthenic move as a stroke of brilliance. It's not about reps; it's about orchestrating a symphony of strength, agility, and flexibility. Calisthenics isn't a routine; it's a lifestyle. And the best part? Anyone can join the party, no VIP pass is required.

So, my friend, as we embark on this journey through the universe of calisthenics, get ready for a rollercoaster ride of self-discovery, strength-building, and maybe a bit of sweating (okay, maybe a lot). This chapter is just the beginning – the warm-up if you will. Ready to redefine your fitness journey? Let's get started!

Why Calisthenics?

In the realm of fitness, amidst the cacophony of workout trends and gym fads, there's one method that stands out like a beacon of functional strength and versatility: Calisthenics. Let's unravel the reasons why calisthenics isn't just a workout; it's a lifestyle, a philosophy, and a transformative journey for your body and mind.

Advantages for Weight Loss:

Calisthenics, with its emphasis on full-body movements and high-intensity workouts, is a powerhouse when it comes to shedding those extra pounds. Picture this: you're not just burning calories during the workout; your body becomes a fat-burning furnace hours after. It's the gift that keeps on giving, helping you torch fat and unveil the lean, sculpted physique you've been dreaming of.

But it's not just about the numbers on the scale. Calisthenics, with its dynamic movements, engages multiple muscle groups simultaneously, revving up your metabolism and turning your body into a finely tuned calorie-burning machine. It's not a crash diet; it's a sustainable, enjoyable approach to weight management.

Muscle Building Mastery:

Now, let's talk muscles, not just any muscles, but lean, functional muscle that empowers you in every aspect of life. Calisthenics, with its focus on bodyweight resistance, promotes balanced muscle development, enhancing both strength and flexibility. Forget about the monotony of isolated weightlifting; calisthenics encourages a symphony of muscle engagement, creating a physique that's not only powerful but agile.

Think about it, every pushup, pullup, and squat isn't just sculpting your body; it's cultivating real-world strength. Calisthenics is about mastering your body in space, creating a harmony between strength and mobility that extends beyond the gym. Say goodbye to the myth that bodyweight training can't pack on muscle – calisthenics enthusiasts are walking proof that it absolutely can.

Overall Fitness Redefined:

Calisthenics isn't just about looking good; it's about feeling good, too. This approach to fitness doesn't compartmentalize health, it integrates strength, endurance, flexibility, and cardiovascular fitness into one seamless package. As you progress in calisthenics, you'll notice improvements in your posture, balance, and overall physical functionality.

It's not a quick fix; it's a holistic approach to well-being. Calisthenics is a lifelong journey that adapts to your fitness level, evolving as you grow stronger and more resilient. You're not just getting fit; you're cultivating a sustainable, adaptable lifestyle that enhances your quality of life.

Addressing Common Misconceptions:

Now, let's dispel a few myths. Some might see calisthenics as suitable only for the super-fit or those chasing Instagram-worthy handstand pushups. In reality, calisthenics is for everyone, from beginners taking their first steps on the fitness journey to seasoned athletes craving a new challenge.

Another misconception revolves around the idea that bodyweight exercises can't deliver the same results as lifting heavy weights. It's time to break free from that mindset. Calisthenics, when approached strategically, can build impressive strength and muscle mass, proving that your body is a powerful tool for transformation.

So, why calisthenics? It's not just a workout; it's a holistic approach to fitness that transcends the limitations of conventional exercise. It's about unlocking the potential within you, sculpting a body that moves with grace and strength, and embracing a lifestyle that goes beyond the walls of the gym. Welcome to the world of calisthenics, where the ordinary becomes extraordinary, and the journey is as transformative as the results.

Chapter 2
Getting Started
Preparation and Goal Setting

Congratulations on taking the first step toward a stronger, more resilient you! In this chapter, we're delving into the nitty-gritty of getting started with calisthenics. It's not just a workout; it's a journey, and like any adventure, a proper beginning sets the tone for success. So, let's lace up those metaphorical sneakers and dive into the essentials of preparing for your calisthenics journey.

Assessing Current Fitness Levels

Alright, let's be real for a moment. Whether you're a seasoned gym-goer or someone whose idea of exercise is reaching for the remote, everyone starts somewhere. The key is understanding where that starting line is for you. In this section, we'll guide you through a self-assessment process to gauge your current fitness levels.

Consider it a friendly fitness checkpoint. We're not here to judge; we're here to understand. You'll discover your strengths, identify areas for improvement, and set a benchmark for your calisthenics journey. No need for fancy gadgets or complex measurements – just a willingness to be honest with yourself and a commitment to progress.

Now that we've laid the groundwork, let's talk about goals. Setting realistic, achievable objectives is the compass that guides your calisthenics adventure. In this section, we'll help you navigate the goal-setting process, ensuring that your aspirations are challenging yet attainable.

It's not just about saying, "I want to get fit." We'll work together to define what "fit" means for you. Whether it's conquering your first pull-up, mastering a flawless pushup, or simply improving your overall stamina, your goals will become the roadmap for your journey. But here's the catch, they're not set in stone. As you progress, your goals will evolve, aligning with your newfound strength and capabilities.

Remember, this isn't about a race to the finish line; it's about enjoying the scenic route, celebrating the small victories, and reveling in the transformation – both physical and mental.

So, grab a pen, a notepad, and maybe a cup of your favorite beverage. In the following pages, we'll guide you through the steps of assessing where you are, envisioning where you want to be, and creating a roadmap to get there. Your calisthenics journey awaits, let's make those first steps count!

Equipment Guide

Welcome to the equipment guide, where we're breaking down the essentials you need to turn your space into a dynamic calisthenics arena. Calisthenics is all about using your body as the gym, but a few key tools can elevate your workout, adding variety and challenge to your routine. In this chapter, we'll explore the must-haves for your calisthenics toolkit.

Essential Equipment for Calisthenics

Bodyweight is the Foundation:

First things first – your body is the primary piece of equipment. It's the barbell, the dumbbell, and the resistance all rolled into one. Calisthenics is the art of mastering your body in motion, and it requires no more than your sheer determination. So, consider this your reminder: whether you're in a spacious gym or a cozy living room, your body is the ultimate workout machine.

Pull-Up Bar:

Meet your new best friend in the calisthenics world – the pull-up bar. This simple yet versatile piece of equipment opens the door to a plethora of upper-body exercises. From pull-ups to hanging leg raises, a sturdy pull-up bar provides the anchor for your vertical conquests.

Parallel Bars/Dip Station:

Ready to target those triceps and chest muscles? Enter the parallel bars or dip station. This piece of equipment is your go-to for dips, leg raises, and a variety of advanced exercises that take your calisthenics routine to new heights literally.

Resistance Bands:

If versatility had a symbol, it would be the resistance band. These stretchy wonders add resistance to your bodyweight exercises, making them more challenging and effective. Whether you're a beginner looking for assistance or an advanced practitioner craving extra resistance, resistance bands are a game-changer.

Exercise Mat:

Comfort matters, especially when you're engaging in ground-based exercises like planks, push-ups, and stretches. An exercise mat provides the cushioning and stability you need, turning any surface into a comfortable workout space.

Optional Add-ons:

While the above are the essential players, feel free to explore optional add-ons like gymnastic rings, a stability ball, or parallettes for an extra layer of diversity in your workouts. These additions can enhance your calisthenics repertoire, keeping your routine exciting and challenging.

Remember, the beauty of calisthenics lies in its accessibility. You don't need rows of expensive machines; you just need the right tools to enhance your body's natural capabilities. So, let's dive into the specifics, explore the world of calisthenics equipment, and discover how these simple tools can unleash your full potential. The stage is set – let the bodyweight symphony begin!

Ah, the excitement of building your own calisthenics setup! In this section, we're not just talking about equipment – we're talking about making it work for your wallet. Whether you're on a budget or ready to invest, we've got recommendations that cater to every financial avenue. Let's navigate the world of calisthenics gear with savvy choices for various budgets.

Recommendations for Various Budgets

Thrifty Essentials:

For the budget-conscious enthusiast, fear not – calisthenics doesn't have to break the bank. Start with the fundamentals: a sturdy pull-up bar that can fit into most door frames. Look for budget-friendly options that offer durability without sacrificing safety. If you're feeling ambitious, a set of reliable resistance bands adds versatility to your routine without burning a hole in your pocket.

Mid-Range Marvels:

Ready to level up? In the mid-range budget, consider investing in a quality dip station or parallel bars. These versatile pieces of equipment open up a whole new dimension of exercises, providing a sturdy foundation for your calisthenics journey. Look for options with adjustable heights and solid construction to ensure longevity.

Investment Picks:

If you're all in and ready to make a lasting investment, consider a combination of high-quality equipment. A multipurpose pull-up and dip station combo can offer a comprehensive solution for upper body workouts. Gymnastic rings are another worthy investment, providing a dynamic element to your routines. Additionally, explore durable resistance bands with various resistance levels for a customized experience.

DIY Creativity:

For the crafty individuals, there's always the option of creating your own equipment. A DIY pull-up bar or parallel bars using sturdy materials can be a cost-effective and rewarding project. Just ensure safety and stability are top priorities in your DIY creations.

Remember, the key is to find the sweet spot between functionality, durability, and your budget. Each piece of equipment should align with your fitness goals and cater to your unique preferences. In the following pages, we'll guide you through specific recommendations for each budget category, ensuring that, regardless of your financial landscape, you can kickstart your calisthenics journey with confidence. Let's turn your workout space into a budget-friendly powerhouse – because gains should never be reserved for the elite!

Chapter 3
Exercise Fundamentals
Basic Bodyweight Movements

Welcome to the core of your calisthenics journey – the Exercise Fundamentals chapter. Here, we'll strip down to the essentials, focusing on the building blocks of bodyweight mastery. Think of it as calisthenics 101, where we'll break down the proper form and step-by-step instructions for foundational movements like pushups, squats, lunges, and more. Let's dive in!

Proper Form for Pushups:

Let's start with the pushup – a timeless classic that's more than just a chest workout. Here's the breakdown:

Body Position: Begin in a plank position, hands slightly wider than shoulder-width apart.

Core Engagement: Keep your core tight and your body in a straight line from head to heels.

Elbow Position: Lower your body by bending your elbows, ensuring they're at a 90-degree angle.

Full Extension: Push back up to the starting position, fully extending your arms.

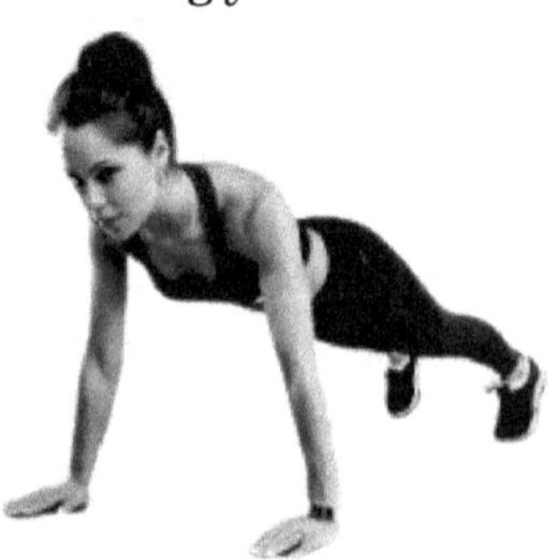

The squat is the king of lower body exercises, and nailing the form is crucial:

Starting Position: Stand with feet shoulder-width apart, toes slightly turned out.

Hips Back: Initiate the movement by pushing your hips back and bending your knees.

Depth: Descend until your thighs are parallel to the ground or as far as your flexibility allows.

Drive Through Heels: Push through your heels to return to the standing position.

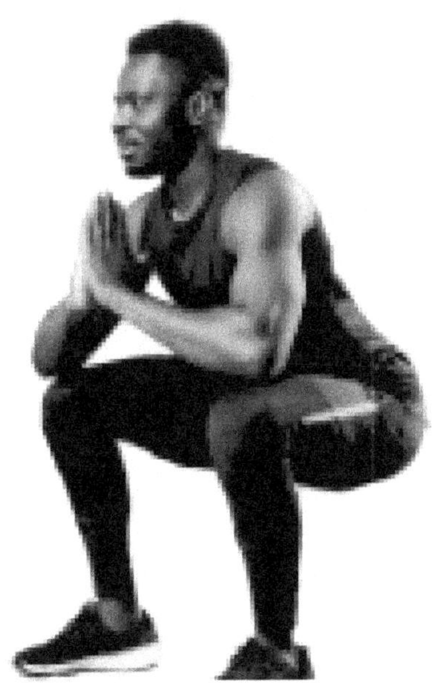

Lunges for Leg Strength:

Lunges are the secret sauce for sculpting those legs and improving balance:

Step Forward: Take a step forward with one leg, lowering your hips until both knees are bent at a 90-degree angle.
Back Knee Hovering: The back knee should hover just above the ground.
Push Back: Push off the front foot to return to the starting position, then repeat on the other leg.

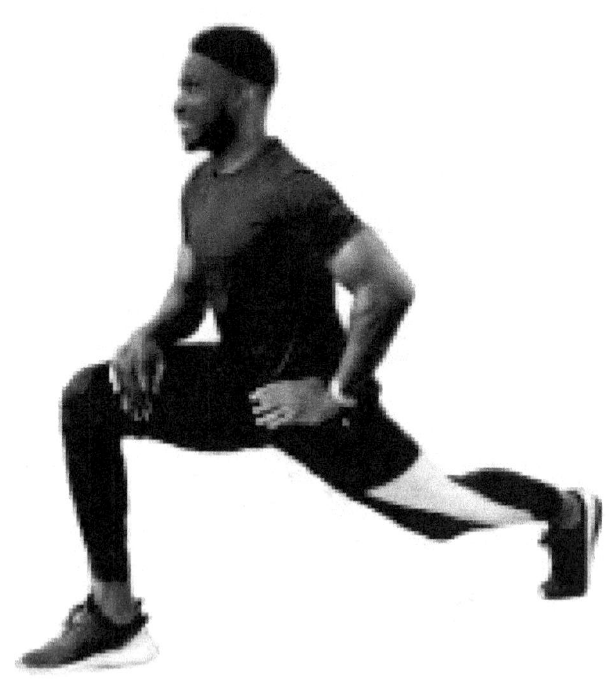

Bodyweight rows are an excellent upper body exercise that targets your back and biceps:

Setup: Find a sturdy horizontal bar or use a suspension trainer.

Body Position: Lie underneath the bar with your heels on the ground, and arms extended.

Pull Up: Pull your chest towards the bar by engaging your back muscles.

Lower with Control: Lower your body back down, maintaining control throughout the movement.

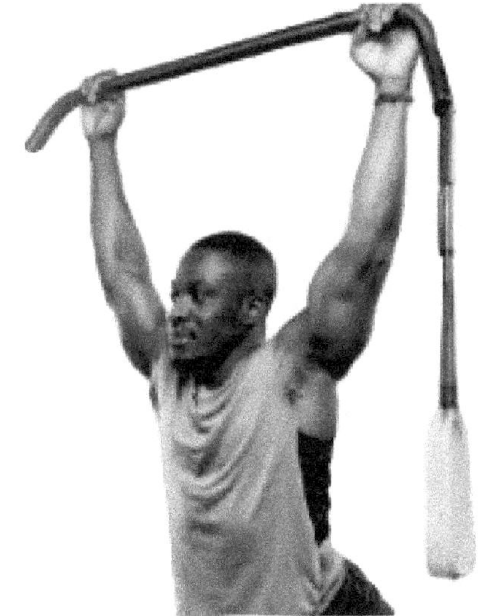

Remember, the devil is in the details. Focus on maintaining proper form, move at a controlled pace, and always prioritize quality over quantity. In the following pages, we'll take a closer look at these fundamental movements, providing detailed instructions, common mistakes to avoid, and tips to maximize effectiveness. It's time to lay the groundwork for a strong and resilient body – let's master these basics together!

Common mistakes and corrections

In our pursuit of mastering the basics in calisthenics, it's crucial to acknowledge that even the most fundamental movements can be marred by common mistakes. Fear not! This chapter is all about shining a light on these pitfalls and providing clear, actionable corrections to keep your form impeccable. Let's dive into the intricacies of each exercise, unraveling the mysteries of common mistakes, and offering the compass to steer you in the right direction.

Pushup Predicaments:

Common Mistake #1: Sagging Hips

Correction: Engage your core to maintain a straight line from head to heels throughout the movement.

Common Mistake #2: Elbows Flaring Out

Correction: Keep your elbows at a 45-degree angle to your torso to protect your shoulder joints.

Squat Slip-Ups:

Common Mistake #1: Leaning Forward

Correction: Sit back into the squat by pushing your hips back, maintaining an upright chest.

Common Mistake #2: Collapsing Knees Inward

Correction: Ensure your knees track in line with your toes to prevent unnecessary stress on the joints.

Common Mistake #1: Shallow Lunges

Correction: Aim for a 90-degree bend in both knees to maximize muscle engagement.

Common Mistake #2: Losing Balance

Correction: Focus on a controlled descent and engage your core for stability.

Bodyweight Row Blunders:

Common Mistake #1: Using Momentum

Correction: Pull your chest towards the bar using your back muscles, avoiding excessive swinging.

Common Mistake #2: Incorrect Hand Placement

Correction: Keep your hands at shoulder-width apart and maintain a neutral wrist position.

These common mistakes are not roadblocks; they're detours waiting to be corrected. As you progress through your calisthenics journey, use this section as your troubleshooting guide. Remember, quality always trumps quantity. Each correction is a stepping stone toward refining your form, preventing injuries, and ensuring optimal effectiveness.

In the following pages, we'll delve deeper into these pitfalls, offering insights into why they occur, how to identify them, and most importantly, how to rectify them. Let's turn these mistakes into opportunities for growth, making each repetition a step toward mastery.

Progressions and Regressions

In the grand tapestry of calisthenics, we recognize that every journey is unique. Enter the world of progressions and regressions, the tools that allow you to tailor your calisthenics routine to your current fitness level and aspirations. In this chapter, we'll unveil the art of gradual advancements and gentle regressions, ensuring that no matter where you are on your fitness journey, calisthenics can meet you there.

Progressions: Elevating Your Challenge:

1. Pushup Progressions:

Beginner: Wall pushups - Start by performing pushups with your hands against a wall, gradually decreasing the angle as you progress.

Intermediate: Knee pushups - Lower the difficulty by performing pushups with your knees on the ground.

Advanced: One-arm pushups - Gradually shift to single-arm pushups for an added challenge.

2. Squat Progressions:

Beginner: Chair squats - Use a chair for support, gradually reducing assistance.

Intermediate: Bodyweight squats - Perform a standard squat with proper form.

Advanced: Pistol squats - Elevate your leg for a unilateral challenge.

3. Lunge Progressions:

Beginner: Stationary lunges - Start with stationary lunges before progressing to forward lunges.

Intermediate: Walking lunges - Incorporate forward movement to increase difficulty.

Advanced: Jumping lunges - Add a dynamic element by incorporating a jump between lunges.

4. Bodyweight Row Progressions:

Beginner: Incline bodyweight rows - Start at a higher angle to reduce resistance.

Intermediate: Horizontal bodyweight rows - Gradually lower the bar or use a lower anchor point.

Advanced: One-arm bodyweight rows - Increase difficulty by pulling with one arm.

Regressions: Gentle Modifications for All Levels:

1. Pushup Regressions:

Advanced to Intermediate: Decline pushups - Elevate your feet to increase difficulty.

Intermediate to Beginner: Wall pushups - Start at a higher angle to decrease resistance.

2. Squat Regressions:

Advanced to Intermediate: Single-leg squats - Shift to assisted single-leg squats.

Intermediate to Beginner: Chair squats - Use a chair for support, gradually reducing assistance.

3. Lunge Regressions:

Advanced to Intermediate: Jumping lunges - Simplify by performing stationary lunges.

Intermediate to Beginner: Stationary lunges - Start with stationary lunges before progressing to walking lunges.

4. Bodyweight Row Regressions:

Advanced to Intermediate: One-arm bodyweight rows - Simplify by using both arms.

Intermediate to Beginner: Incline bodyweight rows - Start at a higher angle to decrease resistance.

Modifications for beginners and challenges for advanced users.

In the dynamic landscape of calisthenics, customization is key. This chapter unveils a spectrum of possibilities, catering to both beginners taking their first steps and advanced users seeking the thrill of heightened challenges. From foundational modifications to exhilarating advanced variations, let's explore the nuances that make calisthenics a journey tailored to your unique fitness level.

Modifications for Beginners: Building Foundations:

1. Assisted Pushups:

Setup: Use a resistance band or an incline to provide assistance.

Execution: Follow the standard pushup form, adjusting the assistance level as needed.

Benefits: Builds upper body strength while accommodating beginners.

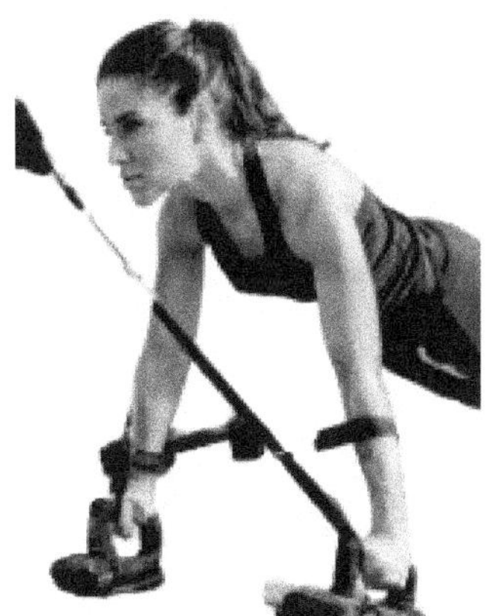

2. Box Squats:

Setup: Stand facing a sturdy box or bench.

Execution: Lower yourself to the box, tapping it lightly before standing up.

Benefits: Simplifies the squat movement while reinforcing proper form.

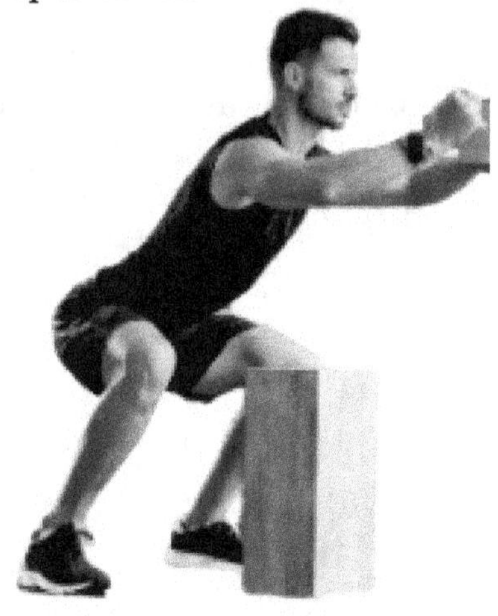

3. Reverse Lunges:

Execution: Step backward with one leg, lowering your body until both knees are at a 90-degree angle.

Benefits: Reduces instability, making lunges more accessible for beginners.

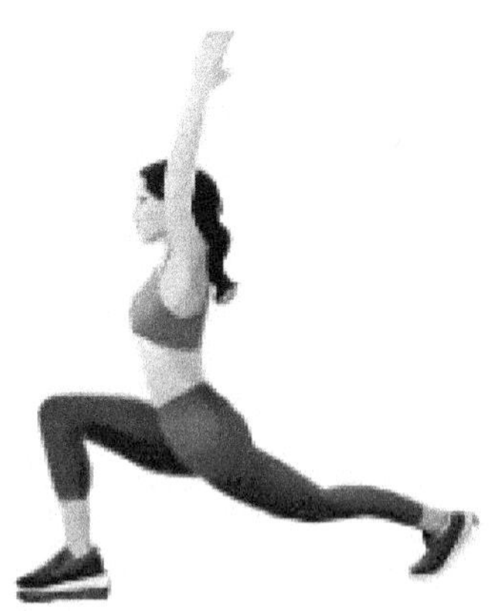

Setup: Use a bar or suspension trainer at hip height.

Execution: Pull your chest toward the bar, keeping your body straight.

Benefits: Establishes a foundation for bodyweight rows.

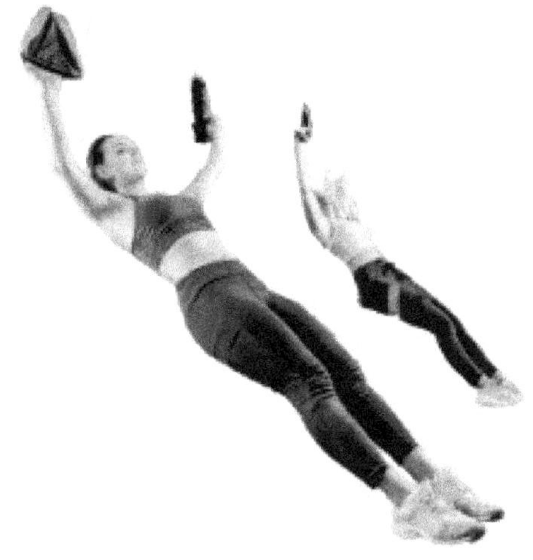

Challenges for Advanced Users: Elevating Intensity

1. Plyometric Pushups:

Execution: Perform explosive pushups, lifting your hands off the ground at the top.

Benefits: Enhances power and explosiveness in the upper body.

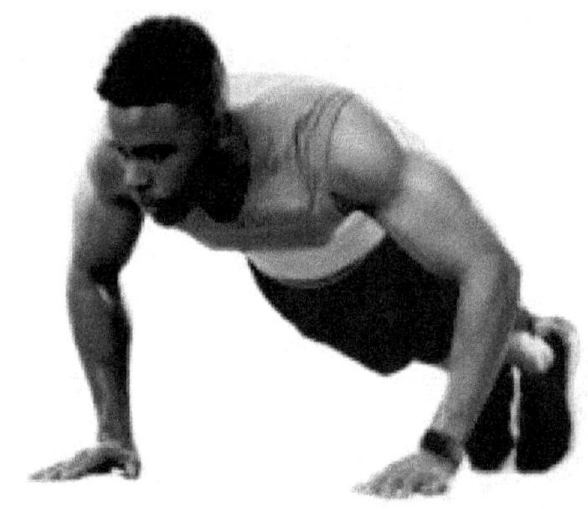

2. Pistol Squats:

Execution: Perform a squat on one leg, lowering your body as far as possible.

Benefits: Requires exceptional strength, balance, and flexibility.

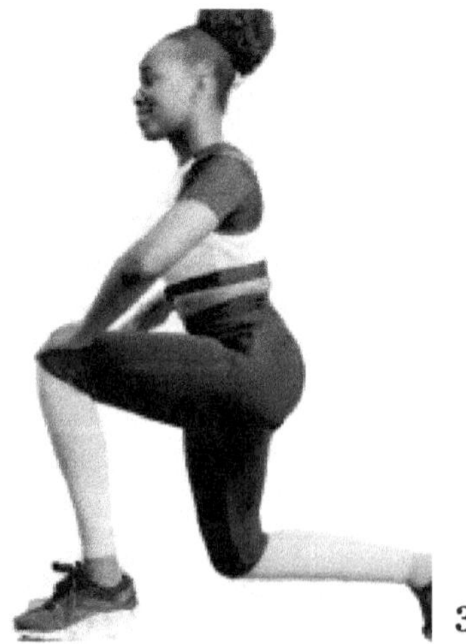

3. Jumping Lunges:

Execution: Alternate between lunging and jumping, switching legs mid-air.
Benefits: Adds a dynamic element, challenging lower body strength and coordination.

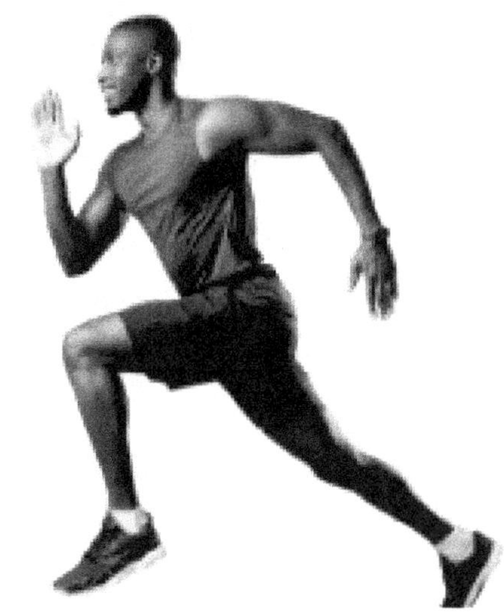

4. Archer Rows:

Execution: Extend one arm fully while pulling with the other during bodyweight rows.
Benefits: Targets each side of the back individually, adding complexity.

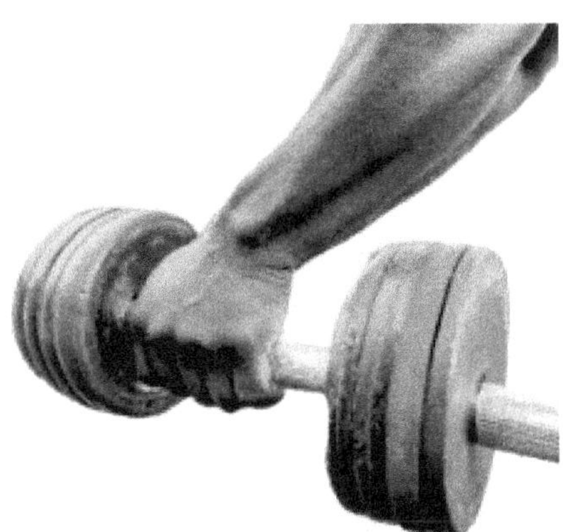

Warm-up and Cool-down Routines

In the realm of calisthenics, success isn't just about the exercises themselves; it's about the journey you take to prepare your body and the care you invest in its recovery. Welcome to the realm of warm-up and cool-down routines, where we unravel the importance of a thorough warm-up, set the stage for peak performance, and pave the way for a serene cool-down that promotes recovery.

Importance of a Thorough Warm-up: Preparing Your Canvas

A warm-up isn't just a prelude; it's your canvas, awaiting the brushstrokes of movement. Here's why a thorough warm-up is non-negotiable:

1. Increased Blood Flow: A proper warm-up enhances blood circulation to your muscles, delivering oxygen and nutrients crucial for optimal performance.

2. Improved Flexibility: Dynamic stretches and joint movements during a warm-up gradually increase flexibility, reducing the risk of injury during exercises.

3. Enhanced Muscle Temperature: Warm muscles contract and relax more efficiently, fostering improved strength and power output.

4. Mental Preparation: Beyond physical benefits, a warm-up mentally readies you for the challenges ahead, sharpening focus and concentration.

Sample Warm-up Routine: Elevating Readiness

1. Cardiovascular Activation:

Activity: Jumping jacks, high knees, or skipping rope.

Duration: 5-7 minutes.

Purpose: Increase heart rate and warm up major muscle groups.

2. Dynamic Stretching:

Activities: Leg swings, arm circles, and torso twists.

Duration: 5-7 minutes.

Purpose: Improve joint flexibility and range of motion.

3. Sport-Specific Movements:

Activity: Light, bodyweight versions of the exercises you'll perform.

Duration: 3-5 minutes.

Purpose: Mimic the upcoming workout, activating targeted muscle groups.

Cool-down Routines: Nurturing Recovery

The final brushstroke in your calisthenics masterpiece is the cool-down, an essential element in ensuring your body transitions gracefully from intense activity to rest and recovery.

1. Decreased Heart Rate:

Activity: Brisk walking or slow jogging.

Duration: 5-7 minutes.

Purpose: Gradually lower heart rate and ease the transition from exercise to rest.

2. Static Stretching:

Activities: Focus on major muscle groups, holding each stretch for 15-30 seconds.

Duration: 7-10 minutes.

Purpose: Enhance flexibility and alleviate muscle tightness.

3. Deep Breathing and Mindfulness:

Activity: Deep diaphragmatic breathing and mindfulness exercises.

Duration: 5 minutes.

Purpose: Encourage relaxation and mental recovery.

In the following pages, we'll delve deeper into the intricacies of warm-up and cool-down routines, offering a holistic understanding of their importance, detailed instructions, and tips for customization. It's time to treat your body with the care it deserves, ensuring not just peak performance but a resilient and thriving physique throughout your calisthenics journey.

Chapter 4
Structuring Your Workouts
Sample Workout Programs

Welcome to the heart of your calisthenics journey, where we lay the foundation for transformative workouts. In this chapter, we'll delve into the art of structuring your workouts, offering sample programs that cater to various fitness goals. Each routine is a carefully composed symphony of movements, designed to elevate your strength, endurance, and overall physical prowess. Let the calisthenics symphony begin!

Full-Body Routine for Strength:

1. Workout Goal: Build Solid Foundations

Warm-up:
- 5-7 minutes of cardiovascular activation (jumping jacks, high knees).
- 5-7 minutes of dynamic stretching (leg swings, arm circles).
- 3-5 minutes of sport-specific movements (bodyweight squats, pushups).

Strength Circuit:
- 3 sets of 8-10 pull-ups.
- 2. Bodyweight Squats: 3 sets of 12-15 reps.
- 3. Pushups: 3 sets of 10-12 reps.
- 4. Inverted Rows: 3 sets of 10-12 reps.

Cooldown:
- Engage in 5-7 minutes of brisk ambulation or light jogging.
- 7-10 minutes of static stretching (hamstrings, chest, back).
- 5 minutes of deep breathing and mindfulness.

Full-Body Routine for Endurance:

2. Workout Goal: Boost Stamina and Cardiovascular Health

Warm-up:
- 7-10 minutes of brisk walking or light jogging.
- 5-7 minutes of dynamic stretching (lunges, arm circles).
- 3-5 minutes of sport-specific movements (jumping jacks, bodyweight rows).

Endurance Circuit:
1. Jumping Lunges: 4 sets of 20 reps (10 per leg).
2. Burpees: 3 sets of 15 reps.
3. Mountain Climbers: 3 sets of 30 seconds.
4. Pushups with Rotation: 3 sets of 12 reps.

Cooldown:
- 7-10 minutes of slow jogging or brisk walking.
- 7-10 minutes of static stretching (quads, calves, shoulders).
- 5 minutes of deep breathing and mindfulness.

Full-Body Routine for Muscle Definition:

3. Workout Goal: Sculpt and Define Muscles

Warm-up:
- 5-7 minutes of light jogging or jumping rope.
- 5-7 minutes of dynamic stretching (leg swings, arm circles).
- 3-5 minutes of sport-specific movements (bodyweight squats, pull-ups).

Definition Circuit:
1. Pistol Squats: 3 sets of 8-10 reps (each leg).
2. Chin-ups: 3 sets of 10-12 reps.
3. Tricep Dips: 3 sets of 15 reps.
4. Plank with Leg Raises: 3 sets of 20 seconds.

Cooldown:
- 5-7 minutes of brisk walking or light jogging.
- 7-10 minutes of static stretching (hamstrings, biceps, triceps).
- 5 minutes of deep breathing and mindfulness.

These sample workout programs serve as blueprints, allowing you to tailor your calisthenics experience to your unique goals. In the upcoming pages, we'll dissect each routine, offering step-by-step instructions, tips for progression, and insights into maximizing effectiveness. Get ready to step onto the stage of your own calisthenics symphony, where every movement is a note, and every workout is a masterpiece in the making.

Fine-Tuning Your Calisthenics Symphony

4. Workout Goal: Flexibility and Mobility Mastery

Warm-up:
- 7-10 minutes of brisk walking combined with dynamic stretches (arm circles, leg swings).
- 3-5 minutes of sport-specific movements (bodyweight squats, lunges).

Flexibility Circuit:
1. Dynamic Lunges: 3 sets of 12 reps (alternating legs).
2. Yoga Pushups: 3 sets of 10 reps.
3. Spiderman Crawls: 3 sets of 20 seconds.
4. Pike Stretch: 3 sets of 15 seconds.

Cooldown:
- 7-10 minutes of slow jogging or brisk walking.
- 10-12 minutes of static stretching focusing on major muscle groups.
- 5 minutes of deep breathing and mindfulness.

Guidelines for Crafting Your Own Workouts:

1. Set Clear Goals:
Define whether you aim to build strength, enhance endurance, sculpt muscles, or improve flexibility.

2. Consider Your Fitness Level:
Tailor the intensity of exercises based on whether you're a beginner, intermediate, or advanced practitioner.

3. Balance Your Routine:
Include exercises targeting different muscle groups to achieve a balanced and functional physique.

4. Progression and Variation:
Gradually increase the difficulty of exercises as you progress, and incorporate variations to keep your routine challenging.

5. Listen to Your Body:
Pay attention to how your body responds to different exercises and adjust your routine accordingly. Rest and recovery are crucial components.

6. Consistency is Key:
Consistent, regular workouts are more effective than sporadic intense sessions. Find a schedule that fits your lifestyle.

7. Enjoy the Journey:
Embrace the process and celebrate small victories. Your calisthenics journey is not just about the destination but the experiences along the way.

In the upcoming pages, we'll delve into the intricacies of each workout program, providing detailed instructions, common pitfalls to avoid, and tips for maximizing effectiveness. Remember, your calisthenics symphony is a personal masterpiece, and each routine is a brushstroke on the canvas of your fitness journey. Get ready to sculpt, define, and elevate your body through the harmonious art of calisthenics. The stage is yours.

How to balance strength and cardio.

In the pursuit of overall fitness and well-being, striking the right balance between strength training and cardiovascular exercise is paramount. This chapter delves into the art of harmonizing these two crucial components of fitness, ensuring that your workout regimen is not only effective but also sustainable in the long run.

Understanding the Dynamics:

1. The Role of Strength Training:
Strength training involves resistance exercises designed to build muscle mass, enhance bone density, and boost overall strength. It often includes bodyweight exercises, weightlifting, or resistance band workouts.

2. The Essence of Cardiovascular Exercise:
Cardio, short for cardiovascular, refers to exercises that elevate your heart rate and enhance your respiratory system's efficiency. Common forms include running, cycling, swimming, and high-intensity interval training (HIIT).

Guidelines for Balance:

1. Define Your Goals:
Understand whether your primary focus is on building muscle and strength or improving cardiovascular endurance. Your goals will shape the emphasis in your workout routine.

2. Incorporate Both Modalities:

A well-rounded fitness regimen should ideally include elements of both strength and cardio. This could mean dedicating specific days to each or combining them within the same session.

3. Create a Balanced Weekly Schedule:

Allocate days for strength training and days for cardiovascular workouts. Consider a split routine, alternating between upper body, lower body, and cardio-focused days.

4. Cardio within Strength Workouts:

Integrate cardiovascular exercises into your strength routine. For instance, between sets of weightlifting, perform activities like jumping jacks, high knees, or jump rope to maintain an elevated heart rate.

5. High-Intensity Interval Training (HIIT):

HIIT combines short bursts of intense exercise with periods of rest or lower-intensity activity. It's an excellent way to incorporate both strength and cardio within a single session, maximizing calorie burn and muscle engagement.

6. Listen to Your Body:

Pay attention to how your body responds to different intensities and volumes of exercise. If you feel fatigued or overly sore, adjust your schedule to allow for proper recovery.

7. Progress Gradually:

As you advance, progressively increase the intensity and duration of your workouts. This applies to both strength and cardio components to avoid plateaus and stimulate ongoing improvements.

Sample Weekly Schedule:

1. Monday:
 - Strength Training (Upper Body Focus)

2. Tuesday:
 - Cardiovascular Exercise (Running, Cycling, or HIIT)

3. Wednesday:
 - Active Recovery (Light cardio, yoga, or mobility work)

4. Thursday:
 - Strength Training (Lower Body Focus)

5. Friday:
 - Cardiovascular Exercise (Swimming, Jump Rope, or HIIT)

6. Saturday:
 - Optional Active Recovery or Light Cardio

7. Sunday:
 - Rest or Gentle Activity (Walking, Stretching)

1. Holistic Fitness:
Balancing strength and cardio promotes comprehensive fitness, enhancing both muscular and cardiovascular health.

2. Effective Weight Management:
Combining strength and cardio optimizes calorie expenditure, aiding in weight management and fat loss.

3. Injury Prevention:
A balanced approach helps prevent overuse injuries associated with repetitive movements in one modality.

4. Sustainable Routine:
Variety and balance make your fitness routine more enjoyable and sustainable in the long term.

As we proceed, we'll explore practical examples, workout routines, and strategies to seamlessly integrate strength and cardio into your fitness regimen. Prepare to embark on a journey that not only transforms your body but also nurtures your overall well-being through the harmonious blend of strength and cardiovascular training.

Adding Intensity: Weighted Calisthenics

In the dynamic world of calisthenics, progression is a constant pursuit. While mastering bodyweight exercises is a significant achievement, the journey doesn't end there. This chapter explores the realm of weighted calisthenics, where the integration of external resistance propels your strength training to new heights. Get ready to embark on a journey that adds a layer of intensity, challenges your muscles in novel ways, and sparks continued progress.

Understanding Weighted Calisthenics:

1. What is Weighted Calisthenics?

Weighted calisthenics involves incorporating additional resistance, typically through the use of weights or weighted accessories, to traditional bodyweight exercises. This adds an extra challenge to your workouts, promoting muscle growth and strength development.

2. Why Integrate Weights?

Weighted calisthenics allows you to continually challenge your muscles as they adapt to bodyweight exercises. It offers a progressive overload, a fundamental principle for muscle growth and strength gains.

Getting Started with Weighted Calisthenics:

1. Selecting Appropriate Weights:

Start with a weight that challenges you but allows you to maintain proper form. This may involve using a weighted vest, dip belt, ankle weights, or other accessories.

2. Choosing the Right Exercises:

Prioritize multi-joint exercises for comprehensive muscular engagement. Classic calisthenics exercises like pull-ups, dips, squats, and pushups can be enhanced with added resistance.

3. Gradual Progression:

Commence with a weight appropriate for your current strength, progressively advancing as progress dictates. Small increments ensure steady progress without compromising form.

4. Maintaining Proper Form:

Maintain precise form for optimal results. Weighted calisthenics can amplify the challenge, so maintaining control is crucial for both effectiveness and safety.

Sample Weighted Calisthenics Routine:

1. Weighted Pull-Ups:
Equipment: Dip belt with a weight plate.
Sets and Reps: 4 sets of 8-10 reps.
Execution: Attach the weight to your dip belt and secure it around your waist. Perform pull-ups with controlled movements.

2. Weighted Dips:
Equipment: Dip belt with a weight plate.
Sets and Reps: 3 sets of 10-12 reps.
Execution: Attach the weight to your dip belt and perform dips, focusing on a full range of motion.

3. Weighted Pistol Squats:
Equipment: Holding a dumbbell or kettlebell.
Sets and Reps: 3 sets of 8-10 reps per leg.
Execution: Hold the weight in front of you and perform pistol squats, maintaining balance and control.

4. Weighted Pushups:
Equipment: Wearing a weighted vest.
Sets and Reps: 4 sets of 12-15 reps.
Execution: Perform pushups with the added resistance of the weighted vest.

Benefits of Weighted Calisthenics:

1. Progressive Overload:
   Adding resistance ensures a progressive overload, challenging your muscles to adapt and grow over time.

2. Strength Plateau Breaker:
   Weighted calisthenics can help break through strength plateaus that may occur with traditional bodyweight exercises.

3. Muscle Hypertrophy:
   The added resistance stimulates muscle growth, leading to increased muscle size and definition.

4. Versatility and Accessibility:
   Weighted calisthenics can be adapted to various fitness levels and easily incorporated into your existing calisthenics routine.

Chapter 5
Nutrition and Diet Tips
Eating for Success

In the intricate dance of calisthenics, the role of nutrition is paramount. This chapter unveils the symbiotic relationship between what you eat and how you perform. Get ready to explore nutritional guidance that complements your calisthenics training, fueling your body for optimal performance, recovery, and overall success.

Understanding the Calisthenics-Nutrition Connection:

1. Fueling the Body:

Proper nutrition serves as the fuel that powers your calisthenics workouts. It provides the energy needed for exercises, supports muscle growth, and aids in recovery.

2. Building Blocks of Success:

Nutrients such as proteins, carbohydrates, fats, vitamins, and minerals are the building blocks of success in calisthenics. Each plays a vital role in sustaining energy levels, enhancing performance, and facilitating recovery.

Guidelines for a Calisthenics-Focused Diet:

1. Balanced Macronutrients:

Ensure a balanced intake of macronutrients – proteins, carbohydrates, and fats. This balance is crucial for energy production, muscle repair, and overall metabolic health.

2. Protein for Muscle Support:

Protein is essential for muscle repair and growth. Incorporate lean sources such as poultry, fish, tofu, beans, and dairy into your diet.

3. Carbohydrates as Energy Fuel:

Carbohydrates are your body's primary energy source. Opt for complex carbohydrates like whole grains, fruits, and vegetables to sustain energy levels during workouts.

4. Healthy Fats for Sustained Energy:

Include sources of healthy fats, such as avocados, nuts, seeds, and olive oil, for sustained energy and overall health.

5. Hydration is Key:

Stay well-hydrated to support proper digestion, nutrient absorption, and overall performance. Water is essential for maintaining optimal body function.

6. Pre-Workout Fuel:

Consume a balanced meal or snack containing carbohydrates and protein about 1-2 hours before your calisthenics workout. This provides sustained energy and supports muscle function.

7. Post-Workout Recovery:

After your workout, prioritize a meal rich in protein and carbohydrates to aid muscle recovery and replenish glycogen stores.

8. Supplements when Necessary:
Consider supplements, such as protein powders or multivitamins, to fill nutritional gaps. However, aim to obtain most of your nutrients from whole foods.

9. Listen to Your Body:
Pay attention to hunger and fullness cues. Eating intuitively ensures you provide your body with what it needs when it needs it.

10. Consistency Over Perfection:
Aim for consistency in your dietary choices rather than striving for perfection. Sustainable habits lead to long-term success.

Sample Calisthenics-Focused Meal Plan:

Breakfast:
- Scrambled eggs with spinach and whole-grain toast.
- Greek yogurt with berries.

Lunch:
- Grilled chicken or tofu salad with mixed greens, quinoa, and a variety of vegetables.
- A piece of fruit.

Snack:
- Nut and seed trail mix.
- Hummus with carrot and cucumber sticks.

Dinner:

- Baked salmon or lentil stew.
- Sweet potato or brown rice.
- Steamed broccoli or mixed vegetables.

Benefits of a Calisthenics-Focused Diet:

1. Optimized Energy Levels:
A well-balanced diet ensures a steady supply of energy for optimal calisthenics performance.

2. Enhanced Muscle Recovery:
Adequate protein and nutrient intake supports muscle repair and recovery post-workout.

3. Improved Endurance and Stamina:
Properly fueled muscles result in improved endurance and stamina during workouts.

4. Sustainable Progress:
Nutrient-dense meals contribute to sustainable progress, helping you achieve long-term calisthenics goals.

Balancing macronutrients and hydration.

In the intricate tapestry of calisthenics training, achieving peak performance is not solely about the exercises you perform but also about how you nourish and hydrate your body. This section explores the critical elements of balancing macronutrients and hydration, offering insights into optimizing your nutritional strategy for sustained energy, muscle support, and overall well-being.

1. Protein: The Muscle Builder

Role in Calisthenics:

Protein is essential for muscle repair, growth, and recovery. During calisthenics training, micro-tears occur in muscle fibers, and adequate protein intake supports the rebuilding process.

Sources:

Incorporate lean protein sources into your diet, such as chicken, turkey, fish, eggs, tofu, legumes, and low-fat dairy products.

Timing:

Distribute protein intake evenly throughout the day, including pre- and post-workout meals to support muscle protein synthesis.

2. Carbohydrates: The Energy Dynamo

Role in Calisthenics:
 Carbohydrates are the body's primary source of energy. They fuel your workouts, support endurance, and replenish glycogen stores after exercise.

Sources:
 Choose complex carbohydrates like whole grains, fruits, vegetables, and legumes for sustained energy release and optimal digestion.

Timing:
 Consume carbohydrates before workouts to provide readily available energy and after workouts to replenish glycogen stores.

3. Fats: The Sustained Energy Source

Role in Calisthenics:
 Healthy fats contribute to overall health, support hormone production, and serve as a source of sustained energy during low to moderate-intensity activities.

Sources:
 Include sources of healthy fats in your diet, such as avocados, nuts, seeds, olive oil, and fatty fish.

Timing:
 Incorporate fats into your meals for a balanced and satiating diet. While not specifically timed around workouts, they contribute to overall energy balance.

1. Meal Composition:
Aim for balanced meals that include a combination of protein, carbohydrates, and fats. This approach promotes sustained energy and satiety.

2. Individualized Needs:
Adjust macronutrient ratios based on your individual needs, goals, and preferences. Consider consulting a nutrition professional for personalized guidance.

3. Periodization:
Adjust macronutrient intake based on your training intensity and goals. Higher carbohydrate intake may be beneficial on intense workout days.

4. Whole Foods Emphasis:
Prioritize whole, nutrient-dense foods over processed options. This ensures a broad spectrum of micronutrients in addition to macronutrients.

5. Experiment and Monitor:
Experiment with different macronutrient ratios and monitor how your body responds. Pay attention to energy levels, recovery, and overall well-being.

Hydration: Quenching the Thirst for Optimal Performance

Importance of Hydration:

1. Regulating Body Temperature:
   Hydration is crucial for regulating body temperature, especially during strenuous calisthenics workouts.

2. Joint Lubrication and Shock Absorption:
   Water acts as a natural lubricant for joints and aids in shock absorption, promoting joint health during dynamic movements.

3. Nutrient Transport:
   Water facilitates the transport of nutrients, ensuring they reach cells efficiently for energy production and muscle repair.

4. Electrolyte Balance:
   Proper hydration helps maintain electrolyte balance, critical for muscle contractions, nerve impulses, and overall cellular function.

Hydration Guidelines for Calisthenics:

1. Pre-Workout Hydration:
   Consume water leading up to your workout to ensure you start in a hydrated state. Aim for at least 16-20 ounces 2-3 hours before exercise.

2. During Exercise:

Sip water throughout your calisthenics session. The American Council on Exercise recommends about 7-10 ounces every 10-20 minutes for moderate-intensity exercise.

3. Post-Workout Hydration:

Rehydrate after exercise to replace fluids lost through sweat. Aim for at least 24 ounces for every pound lost during exercise.

4. Electrolyte Considerations:

If engaging in prolonged or intense exercise, consider sports drinks or electrolyte-infused water to replenish sodium, potassium, and other electrolytes lost through sweat.

5. Thirst as a Guide:

Pay attention to thirst cues. Thirst is a reliable indicator of your body's need for fluid.

6. Environmental Factors:

Adjust fluid intake based on environmental conditions, such as temperature and humidity, which can increase fluid loss through sweat.

Benefits of Optimal Hydration:

1. Enhanced Performance:
   Proper hydration positively influences endurance, strength, and overall performance during calisthenics training.

2. Faster Recovery:
   Adequate hydration supports efficient nutrient transport and enhances the recovery process after exercise.

3. Reduced Risk of Injury:
   Well-hydrated muscles and joints are less prone to injuries, contributing to overall workout safety.

4. Cognitive Function:
   Hydration plays a role in maintaining cognitive function, concentration, and focus during workouts.

As you navigate the intricate balance of macronutrients and hydration, remember that individual needs vary. Tailor your approach based on your unique physiology, training intensity, and personal goals. Consistently fine-tune your nutrition and hydration strategy to optimize your calisthenics performance and foster a resilient, thriving body.

Chapter 6
Mindset and Motivation
Building a Positive Mindset

In the vibrant tapestry of calisthenics, the threads of physical effort and mental fortitude weave together to create a harmonious journey. This chapter explores the intricate interplay of mindset and motivation, illuminating the pivotal role mental resilience plays in achieving and sustaining fitness success. Get ready to embark on a transformative exploration of your inner landscape, discovering the keys to building a positive mindset and staying motivated on your calisthenics journey.

Mindset and Fitness:

1. The Power of Perspective:
   Your mindset shapes your reality. Cultivating a positive outlook fosters a sense of empowerment, resilience, and adaptability in the face of challenges.

2. Overcoming Mental Barriers:
   Calisthenics, like any fitness journey, presents mental challenges. A positive mindset helps overcome self-doubt, fear, and limiting beliefs that may hinder progress.

3. Mind-Body Connection:
   Acknowledging the interconnectedness of mind and body is fundamental. A positive mindset enhances focus, concentration, and the ability to push through physical barriers.

1. Set Realistic Expectations:
   Establish achievable short-term and long-term goals. Celebrate small victories along the way to build confidence and motivation.

2. Cultivate Self-Compassion:
   Be kind to yourself, especially during challenging times. Acknowledge setbacks as part of the journey and learn from them rather than dwelling on perceived failures.

3. Focus on Progress, Not Perfection:
   Embrace the concept of progress over perfection. Each step forward, regardless of size, is a testament to your growth.

4. Positive Affirmations:
   Incorporate positive affirmations into your routine. Remind yourself of your capabilities, strengths, and the progress you've made.

5. Visualization Techniques:
   Visualize success. Picture yourself achieving your fitness goals, feeling the sense of accomplishment, and embodying the strength and vitality you aspire to.

6. Surround Yourself with Positivity:
   Build a support network of individuals who uplift and motivate you. Share your journey with like-minded individuals who understand the challenges and victories.

7. Gratitude Practice:

Cultivate gratitude for your body's abilities and the opportunity to engage in calisthenics. A grateful mindset can shift your focus from perceived limitations to possibilities.

Staying motivated on the journey.

Understanding Motivation:

1. Intrinsic vs. Extrinsic Motivation:
   Intrinsic motivation comes from within, driven by personal enjoyment and satisfaction. Extrinsic motivation involves external factors, such as rewards or recognition.

2. Identifying Personal Drivers:
   Understand what motivates you personally. Is it the joy of movement, the desire for a healthier lifestyle, or the sense of accomplishment? Identify these drivers to sustain motivation.

Strategies for Staying Motivated:

1. Set Clear, Meaningful Goals:
   Define clear, specific goals that align with your values and aspirations. Meaningful objectives provide a powerful source of motivation.

2. Create a Reward System:
   Establish a reward system for achieving milestones. Celebrate your accomplishments with non-food rewards, such as a new workout gear or a day of relaxation.

3. Variety in Workouts:
   Keep your workouts diverse and engaging. Introduce new exercises, routines, or challenges to prevent monotony and reignite motivation.

4. Find Joy in Movement:

Rediscover the joy of movement. Shift the focus from strict performance goals to enjoying the process of physical activity.

5. Accountability Partners:

Partner with someone who shares your fitness goals. Having a workout buddy or an accountability partner can boost motivation and create a sense of camaraderie.

6. Track Progress:

Document your progress, whether through photos, measurements, or journaling. Tangible evidence of your journey serves as a powerful motivator.

7. Reflect on Your Why:

Regularly reflect on the reasons why you started your calisthenics journey. Reconnecting with your initial motivations reinforces your commitment.

8. Adapt and Evolve:

Embrace adaptability. If a particular aspect of your routine becomes monotonous, be open to trying new activities or tweaking your approach.

Overcoming Motivational Challenges:

1. Recognize Burnout Signs:

Be aware of signs of burnout, such as fatigue, lack of interest, or decreased performance. Adjust your routine to allow for adequate rest and recovery.

2. Setbacks as Learning Opportunities:

View setbacks as learning opportunities rather than failures. Use them to refine your approach and strengthen your resilience.

3. Reevaluate and Adjust Goals:

If your initial goals become less motivating, consider reevaluating and setting new, inspiring objectives.

4. Celebrate Consistency:

Recognize the value of consistency. Even on days when motivation wanes, the commitment to staying active contributes to long-term success.

As you navigate the realms of mindset and motivation, remember that both are dynamic, evolving aspects of your fitness journey. Cultivating a positive mindset and staying motivated require ongoing attention and nurturing. Embrace the process, celebrate the journey, and let the synergy of mind and body propel you toward enduring fitness success.

Chapter 7
Avoiding Common Pitfalls
Common Mistakes to Avoid

In the exhilarating world of calisthenics, steering clear of common pitfalls is crucial for a seamless and rewarding experience. This chapter delves into the intricacies of avoiding mistakes that can lead to injuries, setbacks, and plateaus in your calisthenics journey. Prepare to fortify your path with knowledge, resilience, and strategies to overcome challenges along the way.

1. Preventing Injuries and Setbacks:

a. Neglecting Warm-up and Cool-down:

Mistake: Skipping proper warm-up and cool-down routines.

Solution: Prioritize a thorough warm-up to prepare your muscles and joints for exercise. Include dynamic stretches and movements. Implement a cool-down with static stretches to enhance flexibility and aid in recovery.

b. Overtraining:

Mistake: Pushing your body too hard without adequate rest.

Solution: Incorporate rest days into your routine. Listen to your body and adjust intensity and volume accordingly. Overtraining can lead to burnout and increased risk of injuries.

c. Poor Form and Technique:

Mistake: Sacrificing form for quantity, leading to improper technique.

Solution: Prioritize proper form in every exercise. Focus on quality over quantity, ensuring controlled movements for effective and safe training.

d. Ignoring Pain Signals:

Mistake: Ignoring or pushing through pain during workouts.

Solution: Differentiate between discomfort and pain. If an exercise causes sharp or persistent pain, stop and assess. Consult a healthcare professional if needed.

e. Inadequate Recovery:

Mistake: Underestimating the importance of rest and recovery.

Solution: Prioritize sleep, proper nutrition, and active recovery. Allow your body time to repair and adapt to the stress of exercise.

2. Troubleshooting Plateaus:

a. Lack of Progress Tracking:

Mistake: Failing to track and assess your progress.

Solution: Keep a workout journal, take photos, and measure key metrics. Tracking progress helps identify areas for improvement and celebrate achievements.

b. Monotonous Routine:

Mistake: Sticking to the same routine for an extended period.

Solution: Introduce variety into your workouts. Change exercises, modify repetitions and sets, or explore new calisthenics techniques to stimulate muscle growth.

c. Inconsistent Training:

Mistake: Inconsistency in your training schedule.

Solution: Establish a consistent workout routine. Consistency is key for progress. Even on busy days, incorporate short, focused workouts to maintain momentum.

d. Insufficient Challenge:

Mistake: Failing to progressively challenge your body.

Solution: Gradually increase the intensity, difficulty, or duration of your workouts. Challenge your muscles with advanced variations or incorporate weighted calisthenics for continued progress.

e. Emotional Burnout:

Mistake: Allowing burnout to affect your emotional well-being.

Solution: Prioritize mental health. Take breaks when needed, engage in activities you enjoy outside of calisthenics, and foster a balanced lifestyle.

Strategies for a Safe and Progressive Calisthenics Journey

1. Injury Prevention Strategies:

a. Warm-up and Cool-down:

Guidance: Prioritize a comprehensive warm-up and cool-down routine to prepare and recover your muscles.

b. Form Check:

Guidance: Regularly assess and refine your form. Consider recording your workouts to identify areas for improvement.

c. Listen to Your Body:

Guidance: Pay attention to signals of discomfort or pain. If an exercise causes pain, modify or seek professional guidance.

d. Recovery Practices:

Guidance: Implement recovery practices such as active rest, proper nutrition, hydration, and adequate sleep.

2. Overcoming Plateaus:

a. Regular Progress Assessments:

Guidance: Regularly assess your performance, strength, and overall progress to identify areas for improvement.

b. Periodization:

Guidance: Incorporate periodization into your training, alternating between phases of high and low intensity to prevent plateaus.

c. Goal Setting:

Guidance: Set clear, measurable goals and adjust them as you progress. Having specific objectives provides direction and motivation.

d. Cross-Training:

Guidance: Explore other forms of exercise to complement your calisthenics routine. Cross-training can address muscle imbalances and prevent monotony.

e. Mental Well-being:

Guidance: Prioritize mental health. Engage in activities that bring joy, manage stress, and foster a positive mindset to prevent emotional burnout.

By navigating these common pitfalls with awareness and strategic planning, you'll fortify your calisthenics journey against unnecessary setbacks. Embrace the journey with wisdom, resilience, and a commitment to ongoing learning and improvement. Your dedication to a safe and progressive approach will undoubtedly contribute to the longevity and success of your calisthenics adventure.

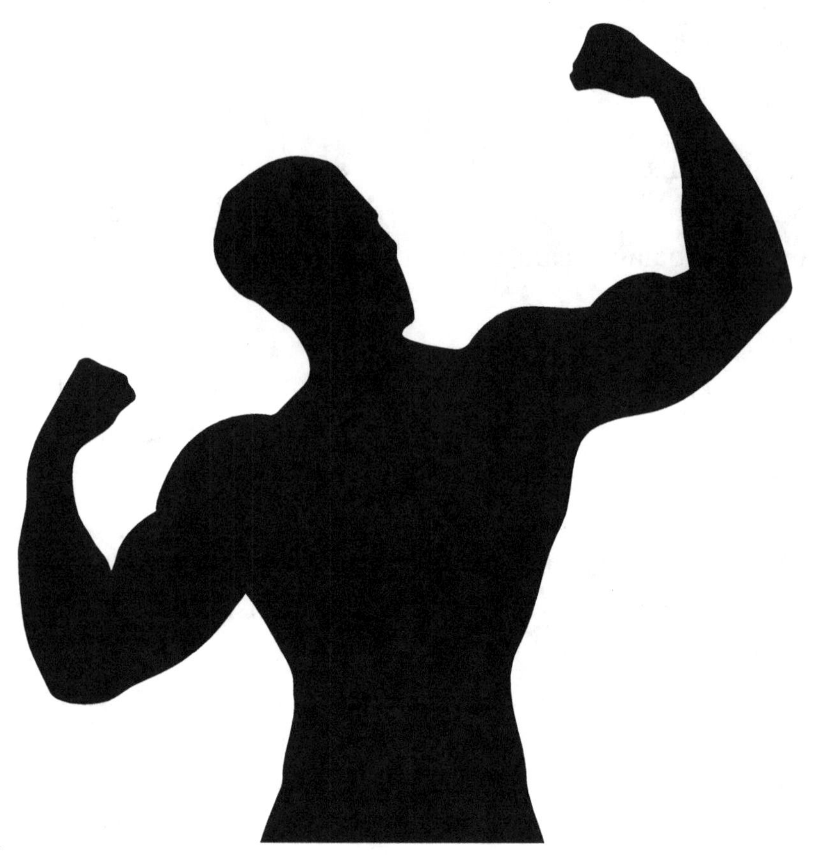

Conclusion

As we reach the final pages of this calisthenics guide, it's not just the conclusion of a book but the beginning of a transformative journey for you – the reader. The chapters within these pages have been crafted with the intention of empowering you with knowledge, guiding you through exercises, and fostering a mindset that transcends the physical aspects of calisthenics.

In your hands, you hold more than just a manual of workouts and routines; you possess a roadmap to a healthier, stronger, and more resilient version of yourself. Calisthenics is not merely about the push-ups, pull-ups, or squats; it's about discovering the depths of your own strength, both physical and mental.

Reflecting on the Path Traveled:

As you reflect on the chapters that have unfolded, remember that every push-up, every progression, and every moment of perseverance contributes to a remarkable narrative – your personal calisthenics journey. The mistakes made and lessons learned are not setbacks but stepping stones towards growth. Your commitment to progress, even in the face of challenges, is the true essence of this endeavor.

Embracing the Mind-Body Connection:

Calisthenics, at its core, is a celebration of the intricate dance between mind and body. The synergy of physical exertion and mental fortitude creates a harmonious rhythm that transcends the boundaries of a workout routine.

This guide has aimed to nurture that connection, reminding you that the strength you cultivate in your muscles is mirrored by the resilience you foster in your mind.

Looking Beyond the Exercises:

Beyond the exercise routines and nutritional guidance lies a philosophy that extends to all facets of life. The principles of discipline, consistency, and adaptability learned on the calisthenics mat are transferable to the broader canvas of your existence. As you carry these principles forward, remember that the journey doesn't end; it evolves.

A Community of Achievers:

You're not alone on this journey. The calisthenics community is a diverse tapestry of individuals, each with their unique stories, goals, and triumphs. Draw inspiration from others, share your experiences, and celebrate the collective spirit of those striving for better versions of themselves.

Your Next Chapter:

As you close this chapter of reading, let it be the prologue to the next phase of your calisthenics adventure. Whether you're a beginner taking the first steps, an enthusiast refining your techniques, or an advanced practitioner seeking new heights, the journey is ongoing.

The pages of your calisthenics story are not bound by the limits of this book. The unwritten chapters await your dedication, resilience, and passion. Approach each workout as a chance to redefine what is possible, each challenge as an opportunity for growth, and each setback as a setup for a greater comeback.

A Grateful Farewell:

It has been a privilege guiding you through these pages. As you embark on the path ahead, may your calisthenics journey be filled with strength, joy, and a profound sense of accomplishment. Farewell for now, and remember – the story of your strength is a tale worth telling, one rep at a time.